GLYCMIC INDEX

A powerful new program for losing
weight and reversing insulin resistance

Sylvia D. Vargas

Table of Contents

CHAPTER 1

THE MINIMIZED GLYCEMIC (MINIMIZED GI) HEALTHY DIETWEIGHT-REDUCTION PLAN METHOD IS ACCORDINGED TO THE IDEA OF THE GLYCEMIC INDEX (GI).

Research observe investigates have genuinely uncovered that the minimized GI healthy diet weight-reduction plan method may also cause fats loss, decrease blood glucose diploma degrees, and decrease the chance of coronary heart hassle and sort 2 diabetic character troubles.

However, the method it positions meals turned into criticized for being unsteady and can't replicate meals` simple healthiness.

These short article substances an in depth compare of the minimized GI healthy diet weight-reduction plan method, containing what it is, approach to abide through it, and its advantages and drawbacks.

Carbohydrates lie in breads, cereals, fruits, veggies,

and milk products. They're a essential a part of a healthful and balanced and additionally stabilized healthy diet weight-reduction plan method.

When you're taking in any kind of kind of kind of carb, your belly device streamlines into very clean sugars that input into the blood stream.

Not all carbs coincide, as unique types have genuinely precise results on blood glucose diploma.

The glycemic index (GI) is a dimension device that positions meals inning conformity with their final results to your blood glucose diploma degrees. It turned into created within side the extraordinarily very early Nineteen Eighties through Dr. David Jenkins, a Canadian educator.

The fees at which unique meals raise blood glucose diploma degrees are ranked then again with the absorption of fifty grams of natural sugar. Pure sugar is used as referral meals and has certainly a GI properly really well worth of one hundred.

- Minimized: fifty five or plenty less
- Device: 56-69
- High: 70 or greater

Foods with a minimized GI properly really well worth are the counseled choice. They're steadily digested and absorbed, growing a slower and smaller sized upward push in blood glucose diploma degrees.

On the unique diverse different hand, meals with a excessive GI properly really well worth have to be limited. They're immediately digested and absorbed, inflicting a fast alternate of blood glucose diploma degrees.

You can use this statistics aid to situate the GI properly really well worth (and glycemic loads, mentioned here) of everyday meals.

It's critical to bear in mind that meals are definitely special a GI properly really well worth in the event that they include carbs. Hence, meals without carbs will now no longer lie on GI statistics. Circumstances of those meals include:

- beef
- chicken
- fish
- eggs
- all-herbal   herbal   herbs
- tastes

SUMMARY

The glycemic index (GI) is a putting device that classifies carb-containing meals through their final results on blood glucose diploma degrees. It turned into created within side the extraordinarily very early Nineteen Eighties through Dr. David Jenkins.

A variety of additives can affect the GI properly really well worth of a meals or recipe, containing:

The kind of sugar it has certainly. There's a wrong concept that sugars have genuinely a excessive GI. The GI of sugar differs from as minimized as 23 for fructose to as excessive as one hundred and five for maltose. As a result, the GI of a meals partially is based at the kind of sugar it has certainly.

The shape of the starch. Starch is a carb manufacturing

up 2 bits — amylose and amylopectin. Amylose is hard to take in, while amylopectin is without difficulty digested. Foods with a better amylose net internet content material will absolutely have genuinely a minimized GI.

Precisely simply how boosted the carb is. Improving techniques which include grinding and rolling prevent amylose and amylopectin bits, raising the GI. Generally chatting, the greater fine-tuned a meals is, the better its GI.

Nourishment framework. Consisting of healthful and balanced healthful protein or fats to a recipe can slow-transferring meals meals digestion and resource in minimizing the glycemic reaction to a recipe.

Cooking method. Preparation performs and cooking strategies can affect the GI additionally. Generally, the plenty longer a meals is ready, the faster its sugars will absolutely be digested and absorbed, raising the GI.

Ripeness. Unripe fruit has certainly made complicated carbs that damages down into sugars because the fruit ripens. The riper the fruit, the better its GI. As an example, an unripe banana has certainly a GI of 30, while an overripe banana has certainly a GI of 48.

SUMMARY

The GI of a meals or recipe is broken through more than a few additives, containing the kind of sugar it has certainly, the shape of the starch, the cooking method, and the extent of ripeness

The value at which meals raise blood glucose diploma degrees is based on three additives: the type of carbs they include, their nourishment framework, and the quantity you're taking in.

However, the GI is a family member determine out that does rule out the quantity of meals taken in. It's often criticized as a result.

To refix this, the glycemic loads (GL) rack up turned into developed.

The GL is a determine out of exactly simply how a carb outcomes blood glucose diploma degrees, taking each the kind (GI) and amount (grams every supplying) into account.

Like the GI, the GL has certainly three classifications:

- Minimized: 10 or plenty less
- Device: 11-19
- High: 20 or greater

The GI remains amongst one of the maximum critical element to remember while adhering to the minimized GI healthy diet weight-reduction plan method.

However, the Glycemic Index Framework, an Australian now no longer-for-income rising comprehending annoying the minimized GI healthy diet weight-reduction plan method, recommends that humans similarly check out their GL and reason to hold their overall everyday GL below one hundred.

Otherwise, the maximum simple method to pick out a GL below one hundred is to select out minimized GI meals while sensible and devour them in little quantities.

The glycemic loads (GL) is a determine out of the kind and amount of the carbs you're taking in. When adhering to the minimized GI healthy dietweight-reduction plan method, it is advocated which you hold your everyday GL below one hundred.

Minimized GI healthy diet weight-reduction plan method and diabetic character troubles

Diabetic character troubles is a complicated sickness that outcomes diverse humans across the globe.

Those which have certainly diabetic character troubles are not able to remedy sugars appropriately, which could make it hard to usually hold healthful and balanced and additionally stabilized blood glucose diploma degrees.

However, superb blood glucose diploma cope with enables live clean of and hold-up the start of troubles, containing coronary heart hassle, stroke, and troubles to the nerves and kidneys.

Could lessen the threat of coronary heart hassle. Existing take a look at studies has without a doubt extraordinarily related excessive GI and GL eating regimen routine applications with a stepped forward threat of coronary heart hassle.

SUMMARY

Minimized GI eating regimen routine applications were related to a discount in weight and cholesterol. On the severa diverse different hand, excessive GI eating regimen routine applications were connected to coronary heart hassle and a stepped forward threat of info cancers cells.

Foods to soak up at the minimized GI eating regimen routine approach

There`s no have to problem energy or tune your healthful and balanced healthful protein, fat, or carbs at the minimized GI eating regimen routine approach.

Instead, the minimized GI eating regimen routine approach includes buying and selling excessive GI meals for minimized GI choices.

There is a top notch deal of healthful and balanced in addition to stabilized and healthful and balanced meals to desire from. You must create your eating regimen routine approach regarding the adhering to minimized GI meals:

- Bread: complete grain, multigrain, rye, sourdough
- Breakfast cereals: metal minimized oats, bran flakes
- Fruit: apples, strawberries, apricots, peaches,

plums, pears, kiwi, tomatoes, and more

- Veggies: carrots, broccoli, cauliflower, celery, zucchini, and more
- Starchy greens: fine potatoes with an orange flesh, corn, yams, wintry weather squash
- Legumes: lentils, chickpeas, baked beans, butter beans, kidney beans, and more
- Pasta and noodles: pasta, soba noodles,

vermicelli noodles, rice noodles

- Rice: basmati, Doongara, considerable grain, brown

- Grains: quinoa, barley, pearl couscous, buckwheat, freekeh, semolina

- Milk and milk substitutes: milk, cheese, yogurt, coconut milk, soy milk, almond milk

The adhering to meals have few or no carbs and as a end result do not have a GI properly worth. These meals can without a doubt be contained as detail of the minimized GI eating regimen routine habitual:

Fish and fish in addition to shellfish: inclusive of salmon, trout, tuna, sardines, and shellfishes

Numerous diverse different animal things: inclusive of red meat, hen, pork, lamb, and eggs

Nuts: along with almonds, cashews, pistachios, walnuts, and macadamia nuts

Fats and oils: inclusive of olive oil, butter, and avocado

All-herbal herbal herbs and tastes: along with garlic, basil, dill, salt, and pepper

To seeking out meals now no longer located in this detailing, outline this records resource.

SUMMARY

The minimized GI eating regimen routine habitual includes switching over excessive GI meals for minimized GI alternatives. For a properly stabilized eating regimen routine habitual, take in minimized GI choices from every of the meals groups.

Foods to keep away from at the minimized GI eating regimen routine habitual

Definitely truly not anything is completely outlawed at the minimized GI eating regimen routine habitual.

Nonetheless, attempt to alter those excessive GI meals with minimized GI alternatives as prolonged as possible:

- Bread: white bread, bagels, naan, Turkish bread, French baguettes, Lebanese bread
- Breakfast cereals: immediately oats, Rice Krispies, Cocoa Krispies, Corn Flakes, Froot Loops
- Starchy greens: Désirée and Red Pontiac potato alternatives, immediately mashed potatoes

- Pasta and noodles: corn pasta and immediately noodles
- Rice: Jasmine, Arborio (utilized in risotto), Calrose, medium-grain white
- Milk substitutes: rice milk and oat milk
- Fruit: watermelon
- Yummy offers with: rice biscuits, Corn Thins, rice cakes, pretzels, corn chips
- Cakes and severa diverse different treats: scones, doughnuts,

cupcakes, cookies, waffles, cakes

- Numerous diverse different: jelly beans, licorice, Gatorade, Lucozade

To keep on with the minimized GI eating regimen routine habitual, restrict your consumption of the excessive GI meals furnished over and rework them with minimized GI alternatives.

An example minimized GI meals desire for 1 week

This example meals desire applications what 1 week at the minimized GI eating regimen routine habitual would possibly seem like. It likewise consists of some of recipes from the Glycemic Index Framework.

Do now no longer be reluctant to alter this or include minimized GI offers with centered to your very own needs and choices.

Monday

- Breakfast: oat dish made with rolled oats, milk, pumpkin seeds, and reduced, fresh, minimized GI fruit

- Lunch: hen sandwich on complete grain bread, supplied with a salad
- Dinner: red meat stir-fry with greens, supplied with considerable grain rice

- Breakfast: complete grain salute with avocado, tomato, and smoked salmon
- Lunch: minestrone soup with an object

of complete grain
bread

- Dinner: barbequed
  fish supplied with
  steamed broccoli and
  inexperienced beans

Wednesday

- Breakfast: omelet
  with mushrooms,
  spinach, tomato, and
  cheese
- Lunch: salmon,
  ricotta, and quinoa
  cups with a salad
- Dinner: self-made
  pizzas made with
  complete wheat
  bread

- Breakfast: smoothie with berries, milk, Greek yogurt, and cinnamon
- Lunch: hen pasta salad made with complete wheat pasta
- Dinner: self-made burgers with red meat patties and greens on complete wheat rolls

- Breakfast: fruity quinoa gruel with apple and cinnamon

- Lunch: toasted tuna salad sandwich on complete wheat bread
- Dinner: hen and chickpea curry with basmati rice

Saturday

- Breakfast: eggs with smoked salmon and tomatoes on complete grain salute
- Lunch: complete grain cowl with egg and lettuce
- Dinner: barbequed lamb chops with environment-

friendlies and
mashed pumpkin

Sunday

- Breakfast:
buckwheat pancakes
with berries

- Lunch: brown rice
and tuna salad

- Dinner: red meat
meatballs supplied
with greens and
brown rice

SUMMARY

The example meal
technique over applications what
1 week at the minimized GI
eating regimen routine habitual
would possibly seem like.

Nonetheless, you could without a doubt rework the technique to healthful your desire and nutritional choices.

Healthy and balanced in addition to stabilized minimized GI offers with

If you discover via way of means of yourself depriving among recipes, accurate indexed underneath are some of healthful and balanced in addition to stabilized minimized GI address standards:

- a handful of unsalted nuts

- a element of fruit with nut butter
- carrot remains with hummus
- a cup of berries or grapes supplied with some of cubes of cheese
- Greek yogurt with sliced almonds
- apple objects with almond butter or peanut butter
- a hard-boiled egg
- minimized GI leftovers from the night time withinside the previous

SUMMARY

Eating offers with among recipes is authorized at the minimized GI eating regimen routine habitual. Some healthful and balanced in addition to stabilized address standards are furnished over.

Downsides of the minimized GI eating regimen routine habitual

Although the minimized GI eating regimen routine habitual has without a doubt surely many benefits, it moreover has without a doubt surely more than a few downsides.

At first, the GI would not provide an ordinary dietary photo. It's critical to moreover don't forget the fat, healthful and balanced healthful protein, sugar, and fiber merchandise of meals, notwithstanding its GI.

As an example, the GI of icy french fries is 75. Some alternatives of baked potato, a loads a great deal more healthy option, have a GI of ninety three or more.

Really, there are a top notch deal of undesirable minimized GI meals, along with a Twix bar (GI 44) and gelato (GI 27-fifty five for slender variants).

CHAPTER 2

GLYCEMIC INDEX OF MEALS

Finding out the GI of meals which you typically devour can actually function if you`re sticking to a minimized glycemic weight loss plan strategy.

Correct indexed underneath are the GI worths for some of elements:

- Fruits
- Apples: 36
- Strawberries: 41
- Days: 42

- Oranges: 43
- Banana: 51
- Mango: 51
- Blueberries: 53
- Pineapple: 59
- Watermelon: 76
- Veggies
- Carrots (boiled): 39
- Plantains (boiled): 66
- Positive potatoes (boiled): 63
- Pumpkin (boiled): 74
- Potatoes (boiled): 78
- Grains
- Barley: 28
- Quinoa: 53

- Rolled oats: fifty five
- Couscous: 65
- Treats: 65
- Brown rice: 68
- White rice: 73
- Whole wheat bread: 74
- White bread: 75
- Legumes
- Soybeans: 16
- Kidney beans: 24
- Chickpeas: 28
- Lentils: 32

Milk matters similarly to exploit options

- Soymilk: 34
- Skim milk: 37
- Whole milk: 39

- Gelato: 51
- Rice milk: 86
- Sweeteners
- Fructose: 15
- Coconut sugar: 54
- Maple syrup: 54
- Honey: 61
- Table sugar: 65

SUMMARY

Acknowledging in which your chosen meals arrived on the glycemic index can actually make it a high-quality deal a lot much less complex to abide through a minimized glycemic weight loss plan strategy.

Without doubt meals, the cooking technique made use can actually impact the glycemic index.

For example, deep-fried meals have the propensity to include a excessive quantity of fats, that may actually slow-transferring the absorption of sugar within side the blood circulate similarly to decrease the GI.

On the diverse different hand, roasting similarly to meals practise can actually damages down immune starch — a kind of starch that takes on meals meals digestion similarly to is usually discovered in meals like legumes, potatoes, similarly to oats — because of this enhancing the GI.

On the diverse different hand, steaming is aspect to do not forget to deliver help guard extra of the immune starch similarly to purpose a minimized GI, in comparison with severa diverse different cooking techniques.

The plenty longer you put together meals like pasta or rice, the lot a long way higher the digestibility in their starch product, similarly to because of this the better their GI. Therefore, it is best to without a doubt put together those meals up until they attain an al dente framework, recommending that they are nevertheless company whilst putting into them.

In addition to the cooking technique made use, the diploma of ripeness may want to moreover impact the GI of a few fruits, containing bananas. This is due to that the quantity of immune starch decreases at some stage in the ripening treatment, growing a better.

For example, bananas which might be absolutely ripened have a GI of 51, while under-ripe bananas have a GI of simply 30.

The diploma of ripeness, similarly to the style in which sure meals are geared up similarly to prepared, can actually impact the GI of entirety item.

CHAPTER 3

WHAT IS THE GLYCEMIC INDEX OF POSITIVE POTATOES?

Positive potatoes are a desired meal valued for his or her preference, versatility, similarly to feasible fitness and well-being and fitness benefits.

Dramatically, cooking techniques have big final results en route your frame digests similarly to absorb them.

While sure strategies may want to have confined end result on blood glucose diploma tiers, others can actually purpose giant spikes similarly to crashes in blood glucose diploma.

This short article topics precisely how the glycemic index of fine potatoes differs relying on precisely how they are geared up.

The glycemic index (GI) is a set up of without a doubt what does it set you back? sure meals enhance blood glucose diploma tiers.

It scores meals on a 0-one hundred range similarly to positions them as minimized, tool, or excessive.

- Minimized: fifty five or plenty a lot much less
- Device: 56-69
- High: 70 or over

Foods excessive in simple carbs or consisted of sugar are harmed down faster within side the blood circulate similarly to have the propensity to have a better GI.

On the diverse different hand, meals excessive in wholesome and balanced wholesome protein, fats, or fiber have plenty a lot much less of a final results on blood glucose diploma tiers similarly to typically a minimized GI.

Various several diverse different variables may want to moreover affect GI properly really well worth, containing meals fragment measurement, enhancing strategies, similarly to cooking techniques.

SUMMARY

The glycemic index (GI) remedies the results that sure meals convey blood glucose diploma tiers. Foods can actually have a minimized, tool, or excessive GI properly really well worth relying on diverse variables.

The style in which meals are geared up can actually have a giant end result at the glycemic index of entirety item. This is mainly real of fine potatoes.

Steaming is notion to regulate the chemical shape of the fine potato, stopping spikes in blood glucose diploma tiers through permitting the starch to be quicker digested through enzymes on your frame.

When steamed, they are moreover notion to guard extra immune starch, a kind of fiber that takes on meals digestion similarly to has clearly in truth a minimized end result on blood glucose diploma tiers.

Steamed fine potatoes have a minimized to tool GI properly really well worth, with a miles higher steaming time lowering the GI.

For example, whilst steamed for 50 percentage a hr, fine potatoes have a minimized GI properly really well worth of referring to 46, but whilst steamed for simply eight minutes, they've a tool GI of 61 (7, eight).

The roasting similarly to meals practice remedies smash immune starch, giving roasted or baked fine potatoes a high-quality deal better glycemic index.

Positive potatoes which have been peeled similarly to roasted have a GI of 82, that's decided as excessive.

Numerous diverse different meals with a comparable GI properly really well worth include rice desserts similarly to activate oat gruel.

Baked fine potatoes have a notably better glycemic index in comparison with diverse different set up.

In truth, fine potatoes which have been peeled similarly to baked for forty five minutes have a GI of 94, production them a excessive-GI meals.

This places them at the very equal diploma with several diverse different excessive-GI meals, containing white rice, baguettes, similarly to activate mashed potatoes.

Deep-fried

Compared with roasted or baked variants, deep-fried fine potatoes have a alternatively lessen glycemic index due to the presence of fats. This is due to that fats can actually hold-up the emptying of the belly similarly to slow-transferring the absorption of sugar within side the blood circulates.

Still, whilst they are deep-fried they've a sensibly excessive GI.

Although the GI properly really well worth can actually range, fine potatoes.

THE END

9 798366 790208